LIFE

HarperCollins*Entertainment*
An Imprint of HarperCollins*Publishers*
77–85 Fulham Palace Road,
Hammersmith, London W6 8JB

www.harpercollins.co.uk

Published by HarperCollins*Entertainment* 2005
1

A catalogue record for this book
is available from the British Library

ISBN 0 00 720135 4

Printed in Belgium by
Proost NV, Turnhout

LIFE

the
INTERESTING
thoughts of
EDWARD
MONKTON

LIVE YOUR DREAMS

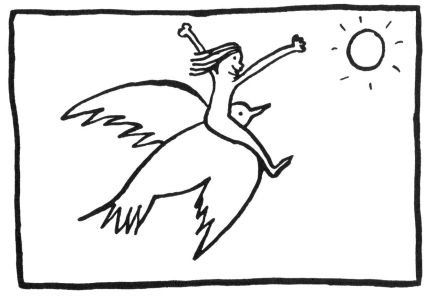

Except for that one about being
EATEN by the GIANT SPIDER

grrr

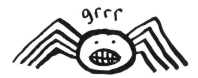

The BEAUTIFUL FROCK

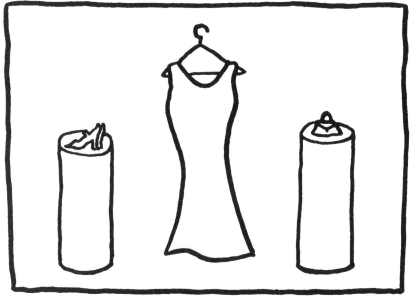

"Buy me, Lady," said the frock, "and I will make you into a BEAUTIFUL and WHOLE and COMPLETE Human Being."

"Do not be SILLY," said the Man, "for a frock alone cannot do that."

"TRUE," said the Lady. "I will have the Shoes and the Bag as well."

The PENGUIN of DEATH

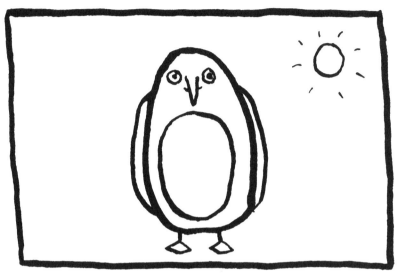

Things you Need to know

1. He is strangely attractive because of his enigmatic smile

2. He can Kill you in any 1 of 412 different ways

THE MEANING of LIFE

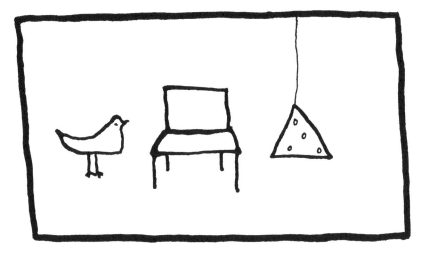

Sometimes it's a chicken
Sometimes it's a chair
Sometimes it's a piece of cheese
Suspended in the air

THE FRIENDS

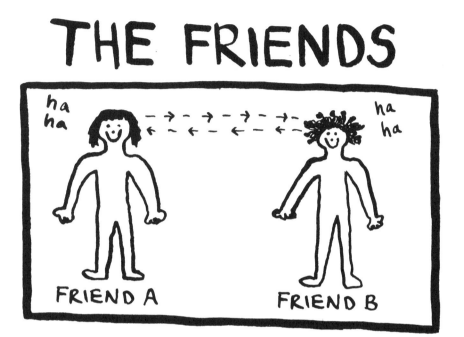

THE FRIENDS can connect in a mysterious way without even speaking.

Perhaps they have AMAZING MAGICAL POWERS.

Perhaps they are both just PECULIAR IN THE HEAD.

LOVE

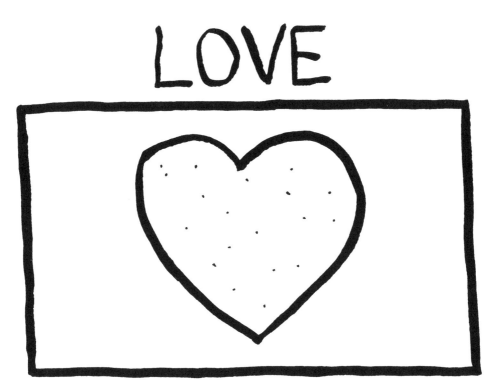

Sometimes the HEART
should FOLLOW the MIND

Sometimes the HEART
should tell the MIND to
STAY AT HOME and
STOP INTERFERING

ARE YOU NORMAL?

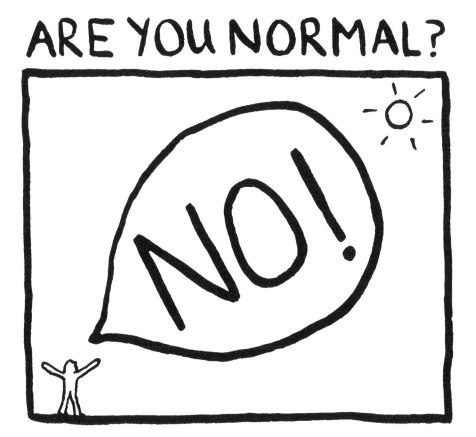

WHERE are we GOING?

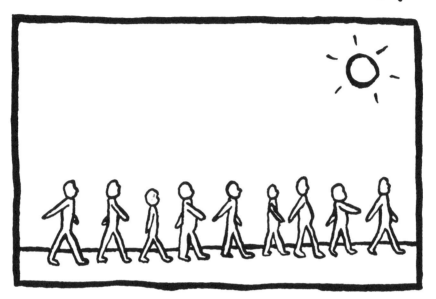

'Where are we going?'
'I don't know. I thought you knew.'
'No, I don't know. Maybe he knows.'
'No. He definitely doesn't know.'

PAUSE

'Maybe no-one knows.'

PAUSE

'oh well. I hope it's nice when we get there.'

MY CHOCOLATE KINGDOM

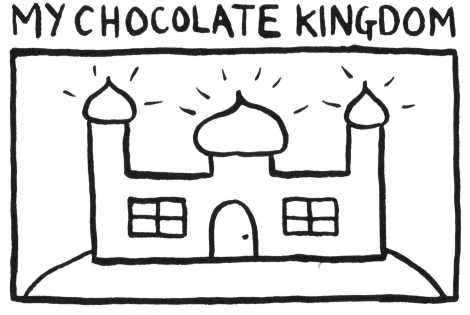

a Fragment of a Dream

... and in my Chocolate Kingdom they brought me great MOUNTAINS of CHOCOLATE and thereof did I eat. And it did not make me feel ILL or ASHAMED, neither did it put weight on my THIGHS. For the chocolate was health-giving and NOURISHING, and the more I ate, the more BEAUTIFUL I became.

The LADY and the SPIDER

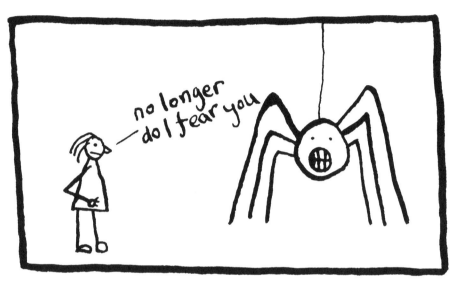

No longer does she fear the
spider. Instead she draws
STRENGTH from the
knowledge of her bravery
in its presence.

YOU ARE LOVELY

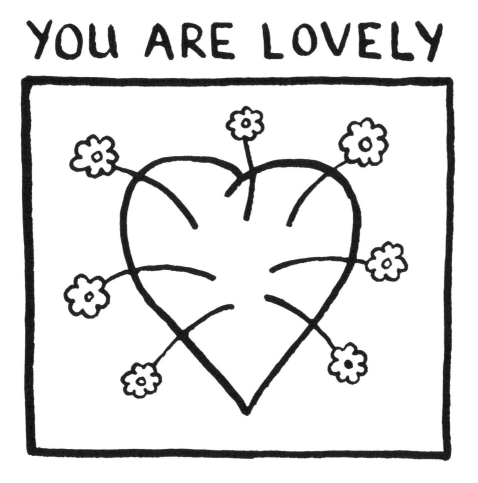

May flowers of HAPPINESS
endlessly GROW in the
sweet ENCHANTED garden
of your HEART

BEAUTIFUL THOUGHTS

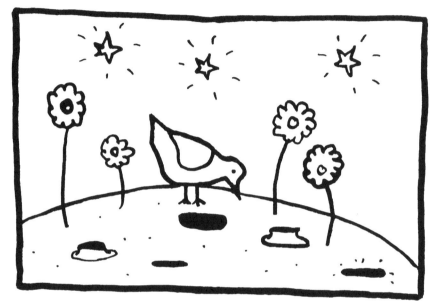

The HOPPY HOPPY SPARROW
plants beautiful thoughts that
grow like FLOWERS in the
BLACKNESS of SPACE

Note

Oh that the World were full of
Hoppy Hoppy Sparrows

NOT ALL POTATOES

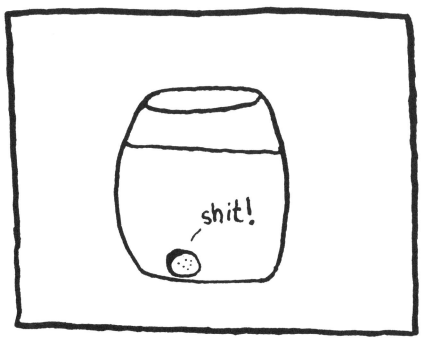

CAN SWIM

GAY SHOPPING

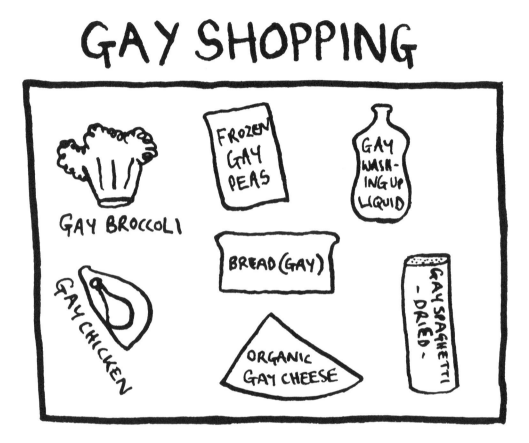

HAPPINESS

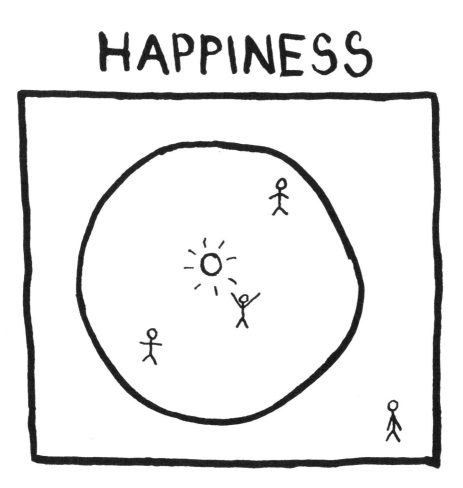

At the centre of the BIG YELLOW CIRCLE
is a TINY GOLDEN DISK. Sometimes
we are VERY NEAR that CENTRE.
Sometimes we are OH SO FAR AWAY.

THINGS to REMEMBER

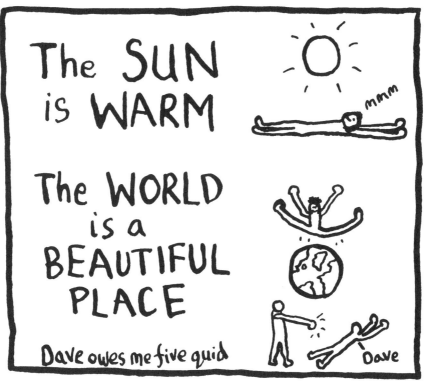

The "MADNESS" hamsters

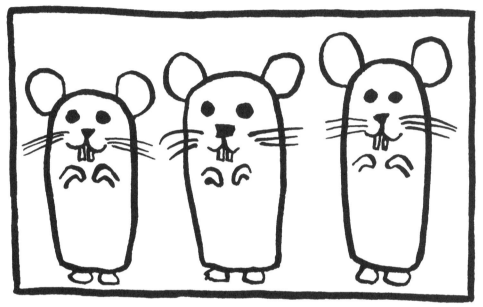

Every night they visit you
Every night they come
And bit by bit
They steal your brain
And feed it to their MUM

THE WONDERFUL GIRL

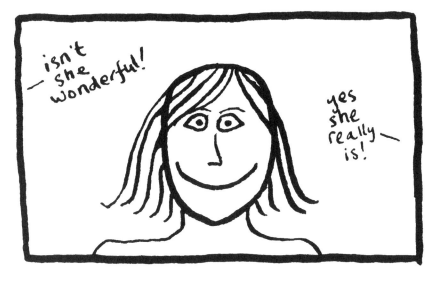

This is a picture of the Wonderful Girl. She is beautiful and STRONG and soft all at the same time.

Everyone who meets her LOVES her and she spreads HAPPINESS wherever she goes.

She is not even frightened of SPIDERS.

INSIGNIFICANT MOMENTS when I have LOVED you with ALL my HEART

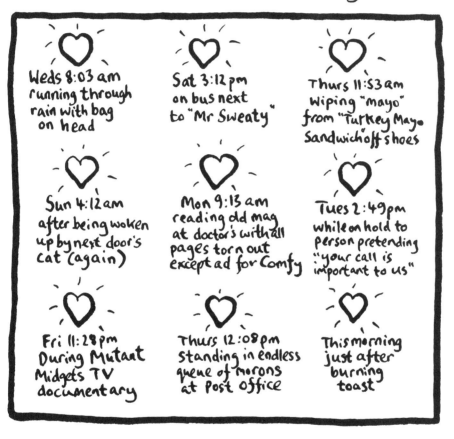

NINJA BISCUITS

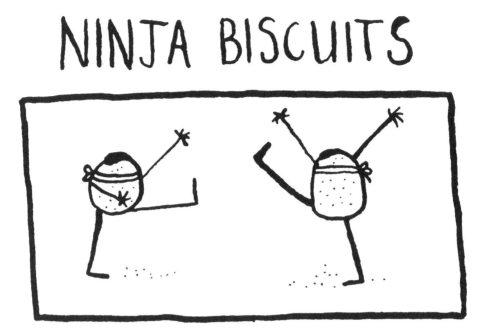

Unfortunately some crumbs
have FALLEN reminding
them of their FRAILTY
in the FACE of TIME

The SHAPES of LOVE

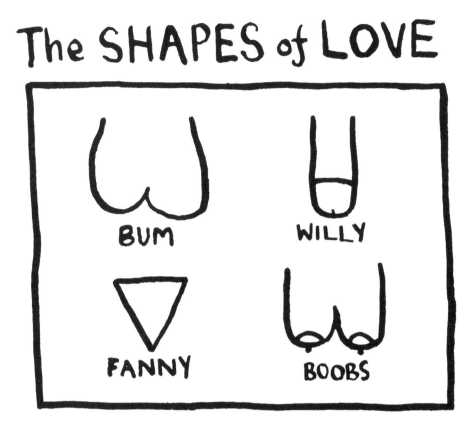

Let us not SNIGGER or be ASHAMED.

Rather let us celebrate the BEAUTY of their SIMPLE PERFECTION.

The HANDBAG of GLORY

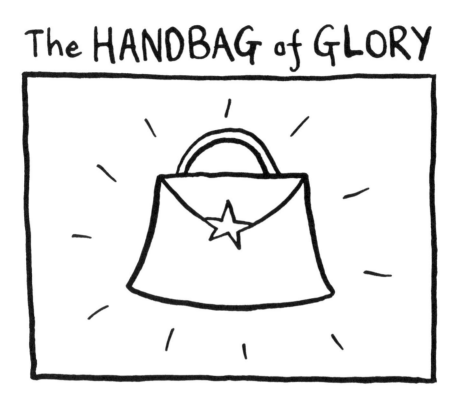

Such was the POWER of the
Handbag of Glory that ladies
WEPT when they saw it and
those who TOUCHED it
went straight to HEAVEN

DEEP THOUGHT

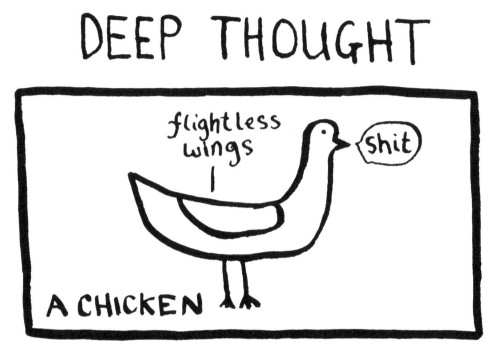

We can all FLY as HIGH as the DREAMS we DARE to LIVE

unless we are a chicken

The Most BEAUTIFUL GIRL in the WORLD

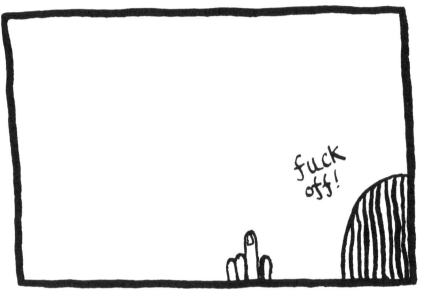

*Unfortunately she spotted my camera and this is the only image I now have of her

FRIENDSHIP

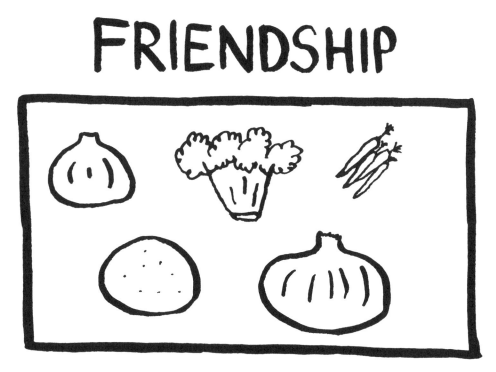

The GARLIC is a friend of the CARROTS
the CARROTS are friends of the POTATO
the ONION is fickle and cannot decide
where her loyalties lie and has hence
formed a **LOVELESS** but **PRACTICAL**
alliance with everyone except the
BROCCOLI. Do not ask about the
BROCCOLI it will only **MAKE YOU CRY**

NICE PEOPLE

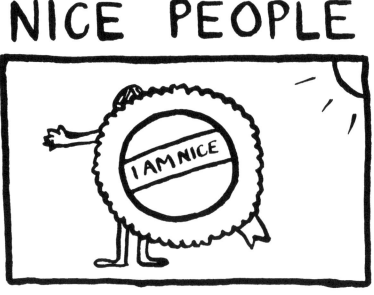

Problem

People who are just **NICE** do not always get **NOTICED**. **NICENESS** is a very **UNDERVALUED** quality.

Solution

The **NICENESS BADGE!!!** *
Of course! Why didn't anyone think of it before ?!!!

* Also we could enter their names in a great book of **NICENESS** that everyone could come and see

The LOVERS

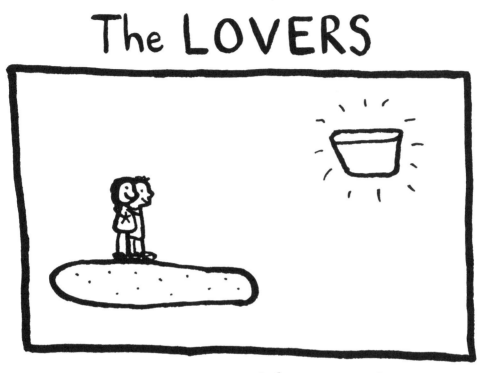

Arm in arm they stand
on the SAUSAGE of LOVE
looking out together at the
KETCHUP of their DREAMS

The POTATO of DOOM

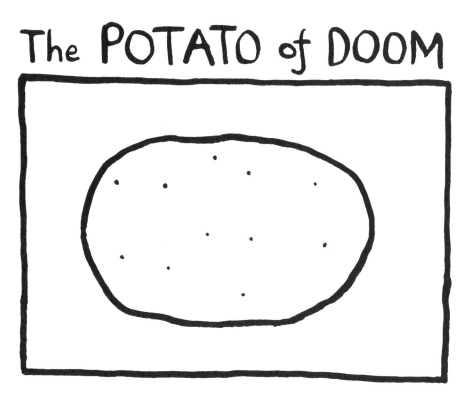

A thousand times it calls your name
A thousand times you hear it
And fools are those who heed its call
Yet fools are those who fear it

We must TAKE our TABLETS or else we will GO MAD

This one helps me not to scare the postman

This one is so BEAUTIFUL it PAINS me to DESTROY it

This one is EVIL and must DIE

I love this one so much it HURTS. One day it will understand my SPECIAL POWERS and love me too

Sometimes I hear this one singing in voices so HAUNTING and LYRICAL that a single note can make me WEEP

"Please don't eat me!"
"Be quiet, tablet, and suffer your FATE!"

The CLOUD of JOY

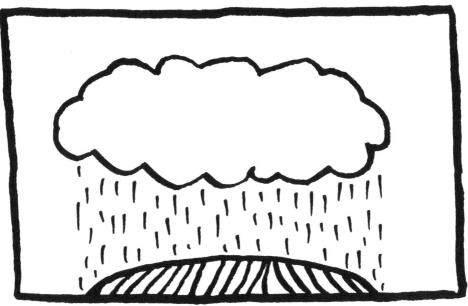

May its gentle RAIN of
HAPPINESS fall soft
upon your head

BEWARE
the TOAST
that has no
EARS!

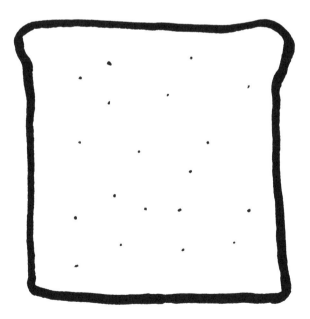

THE PRETTY FLOWERS

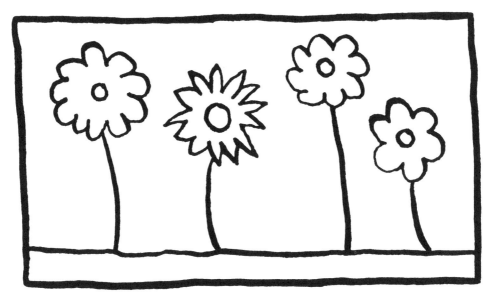

They DANCE not, neither do
they SING, but in their simple
BEAUTY lies more TRUTH
than words are able to express

The HAIRCARE HEDGEHOG

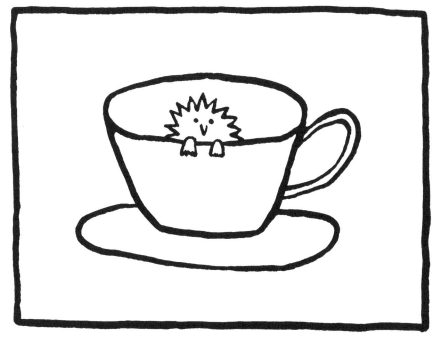

From deep within my cup of tea
The Haircare Hedgehog speaks to me
And tells me with a knowing smile
The secrets of the perfect style

I LOVE YOU

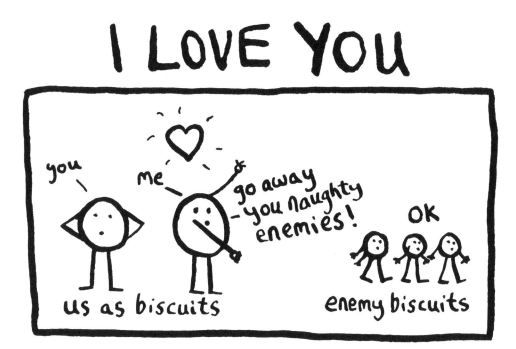

This picture of my DREAM shows how much I LOVE YOU*

* if you are not impressed by the biscuit thing PLEASE remember that it was only a DREAM

LIFE

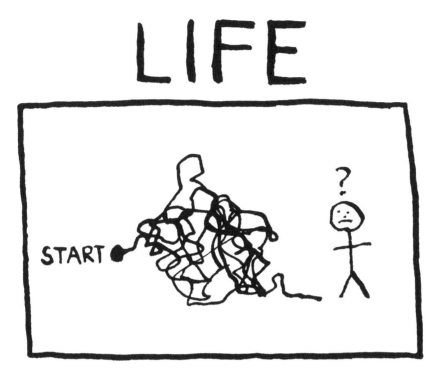

THE END